THE LARYNGECTOMEE GUIDE

FOR COVID -19 PANDEMIC

Itzhak Brook, M.D., M.Sc.

TABLE OF CONTENTS

Introduction……………………………………………………………………………**7**

Chapter 1: Preventing and protecting neck breathers (including laryngectomees) and cancer patients from COVID-19…………………………………………………………**8**

Prevention of Corona virus infection in neck breathers (including laryngectomees)…..8

Signs and symptoms of COVID-19 infection…..13

Information about facemasks, N95 respirator and soft face cover for neck breathers…..14

Beard or facial hair interfere with face mask's efficacy against COVID-19…..16

Protecting immunocompromised patients from COVID-19…..17

Coping with COVID-19 pandemic as head and neck cancer patient…..18

COVID-19 testing in laryngectomees…..20

Chapter 2: Psychological and social issues in head and neck patients (including laryngectomees) caused by the COVID-19 pandemic………………………………………**22**

Mental health issues in head and neck patients (including laryngectomees) caused by the COVID -19 pandemic…..22

Coping with depression…..23

Overcoming depression…..24

How laryngectomees can cope with the COVID -19 quarantine…..26

Going outside during the COVID-19 pandemic. What should laryngectomees do?.....28

How to avoid and cope with quarantine fatigue…..29

Chapter 3. How to take care of voice prosthesis leakage or dislodgement during the corona pandemic…………………………………………………………………………….31

Coping with voice prosthesis leakage or dislodgement during the corona (COVID- 19) pandemic…..31

Cleaning the voice prosthesis and preventing leaking…..33

Maintenance and prevention of leakage…..33

Preventing biofilm of yeast and bacteria from growing on the voice prosthesis…..35

Chapter 4: Mucus, respiratory care, and fitness during the COVID-19 pandemic………..38

Mucus production and increasing air humidity…..38

Respiratory rehabilitation…..39

Keeping fit and eating adequate nutrition during the COVID-19 pandemic…..41

Chapter 5: Treating fibrosis and lymphedema and dealing with esophageal dilation……..43

Fibrosis and lymphedema treatment during the COVID-19 pandemic…..43

How to cope with neopharyngeal or esophageal narrowing during the COVID-19 pandemic…44

Chapter 6: Hospitalization……………………………………………………………..45

Preparing a kit with essential information and material when going to the hospital…..45

Ensuring adequate care during hospitalization for neck breathers including laryngectomees…..47

Chapter 7: Guidelines for head and neck cancer care during COVID-19 pandemic…….51

Head and neck cancer care during COVID-19 pandemic…..51

Chapter 8: Making home Corona virus proof…….………………………………………......54

How to coronavirus-proof your home…..54

Addendum…………………………………………………………………57

Useful resources…..57

Laryngectomees groups in Facebook…..58

List of the major medical suppliers for laryngectomees…..59

About the author………………………………………………………….60

Dedication

The guide is dedicated to my fellow laryngectomees and their caregivers for their courage and perseverance.

Disclaimer

Dr. Brook is not an expert in otolaryngology and head and neck surgery. This guide is not a substitute for medical care by medical professionals.

Introduction

The corona (COVID-19) pandemic presents many medical, social and psychological challenges for laryngectomees and their medical providers. The Laryngectomee Guide for COVID -19 provides information for laryngectomee and neck breathers how to cope with the COVID -19 pandemic. It contains information how to prevent the infection and deal with depression, social isolation, fibrosis, lymphedema, mucous problems, and voice prosthesis leak. It provides suggestions how to deal with esophageal dilation, hospitalization, and keep fit and eat well.

Additional information about laryngectomee care can be found in "The Laryngectomee Guide", "The Laryngectomee Guide Expanded Edition" (both are available as free eBook, paperback and Kindle through Amazon, see page xxx). Similar information is also available at my website "My Voice" (https://dribrook.blogspot.com/). The guides and website contains information about the side effects of radiation and chemotherapy; the methods of speaking after laryngectomy; how to care for the airways, stoma, heat and moisture exchange filter, and voice prosthesis. Additionally they address eating and swallowing issues, medical, dental and psychological concerns, respiration and anesthesia, hospitalization and travelling as a laryngectomee.

The information and advice given in the Laryngectomee Guide for COVID- 19 infection is based on the recommendations and knowledge available at the time of preparing the guide on June 1, 2020. The information and knowledge about the prevention and management of COCID- 19 is growing and constantly evolving. Because the recommendations for COVID- 19 prevention and treatment may change, it is important to follow the local health department and Center of Disease Control and Prevention updates and consulting with medical professionals.

Although this guide is not a substitute for professional medical care, it can be useful for laryngectomees and their caregivers in managing their lives and coping with the challenges of the COVID- 19 pandemic.

Chapter 1:

Preventing and protecting neck breathers (including laryngectomees) and cancer patients from COVID- 19

Prevention of Corona virus infection in neck breathers (including laryngectomees)

Most individuals experience less "colds" after laryngectomy. This is believed to be because respiratory viruses generally first infect the nose before spreading to other body sites (including the lungs). Because laryngectomees do not inhale through their noses this mode of transmission is rare.

However, all respiratory viruses (including COVID-19) can also access the body through the nose, mouth, conjunctiva and stoma (in neck breathers) after they are inhaled or introduced by a contaminated object or hand. It is therefore prudent that laryngectomees are extra vigilant in protecting themselves.

Laryngectomees may also be at risk for poor outcomes with COVID-19 due to other medical comorbidity (e.g., chronic pulmonary disease, peripheral vascular disease, cardiac disease, cerebrovascular disease, diabetes, the underlying cancer history), and the propensity for lower lobs collapse (atelectasis) due to loss of upper airway resistance. Additionally, because many laryngectomees have a smoking history, they are also prone to acute infections due to impaired mucociliary function and mucosal irritation from cold, dry inspired air.

There have been several laryngectomees who acquired COVID-19 infection. Those who were diagnosed had a broad spectrum of symptoms from minimal to severe. There were at least 2 who also had comorbidities that died from COVID-19 infection.

The information and knowledge about the prevention and management of COCID-19 is growing and constantly evolving. Because the recommendations for COVID-19 prevention and treatment may change, it is important to follow the local health department and Center of Disease Control and Prevention (CDC) updates and consulting with medical professionals.

If someone in close contact with laryngectomee is exposed or infected with COVID-19, he / she should self-quarantine themselves and avoid any contact with the neck breather. It is important that laryngectomees protect themselves and others in the community from COVID-19. Due to the increased aerosolization risk from their stoma, the potential to become "super spreaders" necessitates that total laryngectomy patients always cover their stoma in public. The best protection against aerosolization and inhalation of viral particles in the community is to cover the stoma with an HME that includes a bacterial and / or viral filter. Many patients prefer to use laryngectomy tubes, but during this pandemic, an HME attached to the stoma with a baseplate allows for a seal that will force all air through the HME, thus further minimizing aerosolization. If the patient is unable to obtain a good seal with the HME base plate, they can use laryngectomy tubes that accept HME filters is an option.

Laryngectomees can protect themselves and others by taking these steps:

- Wearing heat and moisture exchanger (HME) 24/7 especially when being around other people. HME with greater filtering ability would work better in reducing the risk of inhaling the virus (i.e., Provox MicronTM). (**Picture 1**) Provox Micron, has an electrostatic filter and > 99.9% filtration rate and it's cover prevents direct finger contact with the stoma when speaking. Wearing it also protects other individuals when the laryngectomee is infected. It has maximal activity during the first 24 hours of use. Provox HME Cassette Adapter enables the use of a Provox HME Cassette to any tracheostomy tube with a 15 mm ISO connector. Those with tracheostomy can protect themselves by using ProTrach XtraCare HME .

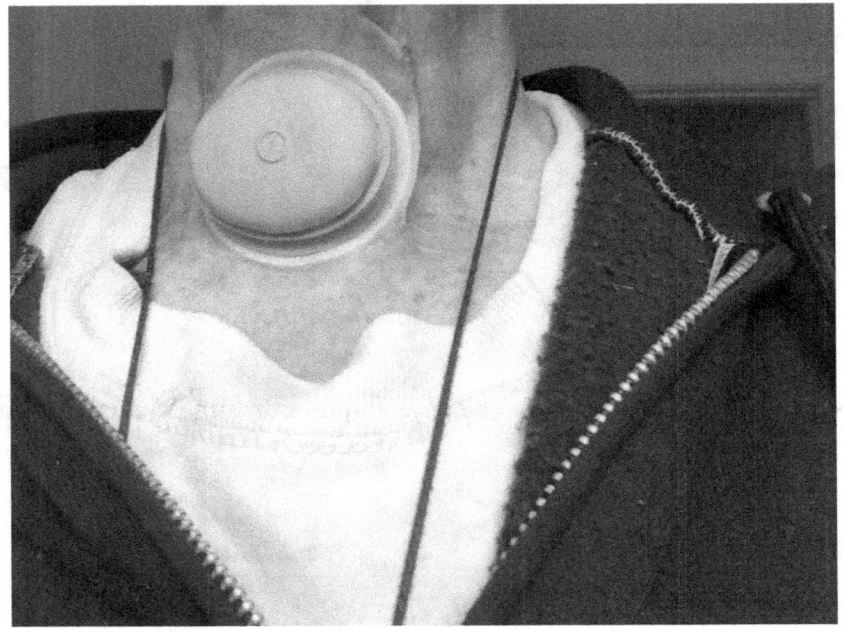

- Wearing hands free tracheostoma valve (because it does not require touching when speaking) in those using trachea esophageal speech. Those who use a regular HME should wash their hands before touching their HME.

- Wearing a surgical mask (**Picture 2, 3**), 100% cotton turtleneck, bib, or scarf over the stoma (in addition to the HME). Tie the upper strings of the mask around neck, use additional extension string to connect the two lower mask strings together under the arms and behind the back. (**Pictures 4-6**)

- Wearing an additional surgical mask or respirator over the nose and mouth, and protective glasses or face shield (**Picture 2, 3**). This can prevent the virus from entering the body through these sites or spread to other people when infected. Men should shave their facial hair prior to wearing surgical mask or respirator. If worn properly, a surgical mask can help block large-particle droplets, splashes, sprays or splatter that may contain microorganism (viruses and bacteria). (**Picture 7**) While a surgical mask may be effective in blocking splashes and large-particle droplets, it does not filter or block very small particles in the air that may be transmitted by coughs, and sneezes. Wearing the mask on the stoma and face also serves in preventing laryngectomees from touching these locations with unclean hands.

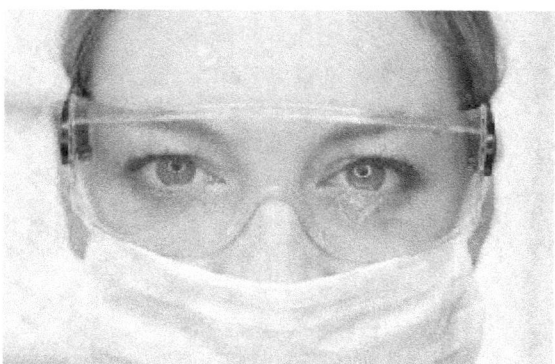

Picture 2: Wearing surgical mask over the nose and mouth, and protective glasses

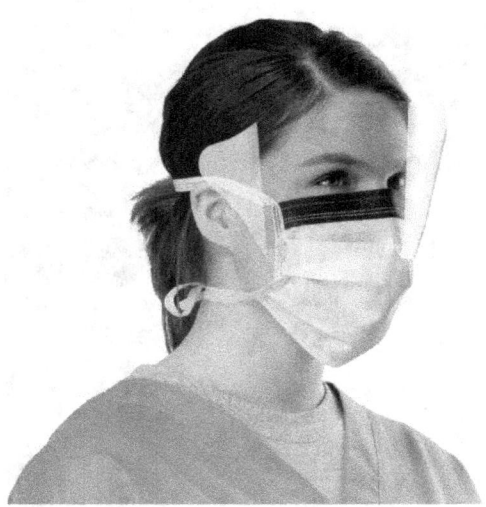

Picture 3: Wearing face shield and surgical mask

- Washing hands often with soap and water for at least 20 seconds. Use an alcohol-based hand sanitizer that contains at least 60% alcohol if soap and water are not available. This is especially important before managing the stoma, and touching the HME when speaking using tracheoesophageal speech.

- Avoiding touching the stoma, HME, eyes, nose, and mouth with unwashed hands. A useful routine is to use the non-dominant hand to touch the stoma and the dominant hand for other activities (e.g., touching a door handle).

- Avoiding close contact with sick people and avoid public and crowded places.

- Cleaning and disinfecting frequently touched objects and surfaces.

Those in close contact with neck breathers can expose them to the virus when they become asymptomatic carrier or infected with COVID-19. These individuals as well as the neck breathers should observe meticulous hand hygiene and wear surgical masks, gloves, eye shields, and other protective items whenever they are in contact with each other.

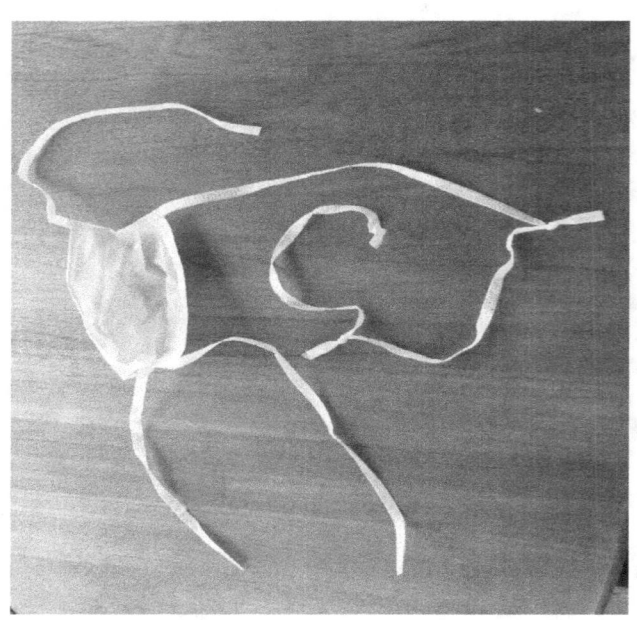

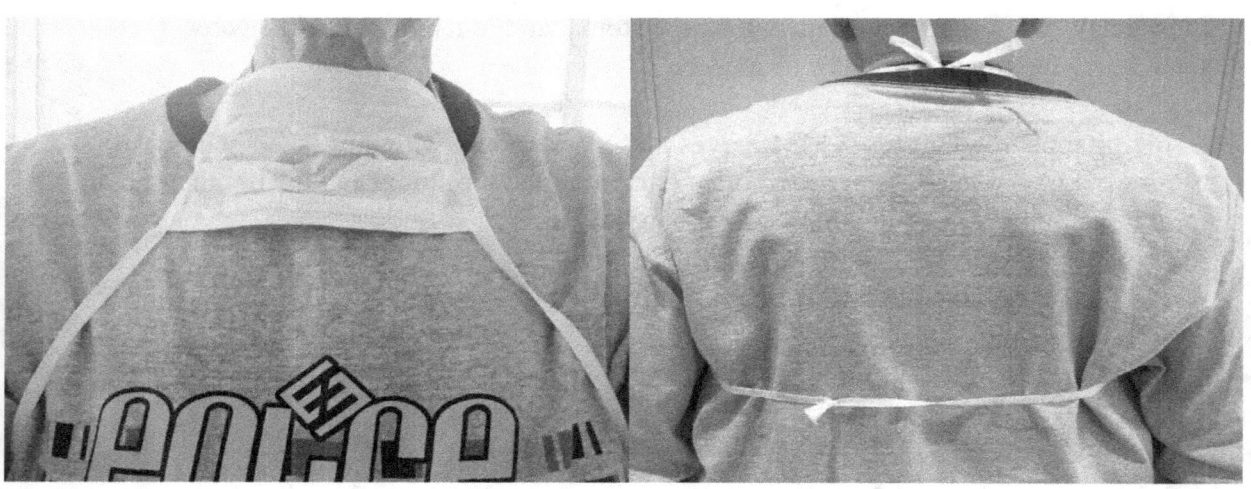

Pictures 4-6: Wearing a modified face mask over the stoma

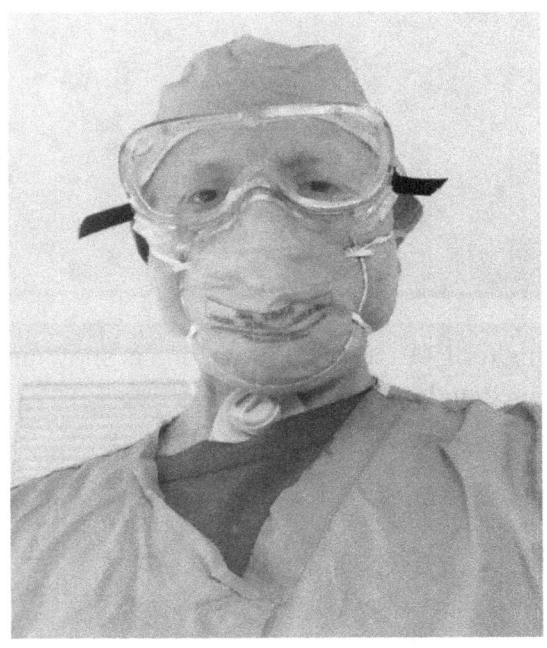

Picture 7: Protection using Provox Micron, N95 face mask and protective glasses.

Further reading about protection of laryngectomees (Oral Oncolgy editorial April, 2020 at: https://www.ncbi.nlm.nih.gov/pmc/articles/PMC7180359/pdf/main.pdf

Signs and symptoms of COVID-19 infection

COVID-19 affects different people in different ways. Infected people have had a wide range of symptoms reported – from mild symptoms to severe illness.

Symptoms may appear 2-14 days after exposure to the virus. The CDC recommends that people with these symptoms may have COVID-19 https://www.cdc.gov/coronavirus/2019-ncov/symptoms-testing/symptoms.html):

- Fever or chills
- Cough
- Shortness of breath or difficulty breathing
- Fatigue
- Muscle or body aches

- Headache
- New loss of taste or smell
- Sore throat
- Congestion or runny nose
- Nausea or vomiting
- Diarrhea

Look for emergency warning signs for COVID-19. If someone is showing any of these signs, seek emergency medical care immediately:

- Trouble breathing
- Persistent pain or pressure in the chest
- New confusion
- Inability to wake or stay awake
- Bluish lips or face

Call your medical provider for any other symptoms that are severe or concerning to you.

Information about facemasks, N95 respirator and soft face cover for neck breathers

It is recommended that neck breathers including laryngectomees cover their stoma (even when using an HME) and nose and mouth with two surgical masks or respirator (stoma only), and if these are not available with a soft (cloth) cover.

If worn properly, a surgical mask can help block large-particle droplets, splashes, sprays or splatter that may contain germs (viruses and bacteria). Surgical masks may also help reduce exposure of the wearer's respiratory secretions to others.

While a surgical mask may be effective in blocking splashes and large-particle droplets, it does not filter or block very small particles in the air that may be transmitted by coughs, and sneezes. It is important to note that the use of an N95 respirator and face shield may not be 100% effective at preventing COVID-19 transmission. Two recent meta-analyses; by Smith et al., and Long et al, failed to demonstrate the superiority of N95 respirators over standard surgical masks in preventing influenza.

An N95 respirator (the "N" means Not effective against oily materials, the "95" means 95% of non-oily airborne particles are filtered out, and the "respirator" means a device that protects against inhalation of hazardous particles) works by providing both a physical and an electrostatic barrier to incoming droplets carrying SARS-CoV-2 virus particles. (**Picture 8**) They are 95%

effective at filtering out particles larger than 0.3 microns. Although the virus particles themselves are smaller than 0.2 microns, they are carried by much larger droplets of water, mucus, and saliva. Because the pores in the respirators are about 1 micron in size, the electrostatic component of filtration is very important in providing protection.

The outer layer of the N95 mask is made of fluid-resistant material to keep moisture from coming in, and the inner layer is made of synthetic fabric. When washed with soap and water, it loses much of its efficiency. UV light and H_2O_2 fumes as well as warm, moist heat destroy the viruses without damaging the synthetic fabric and may permit reuse without diminishing efficiency.

If a respirator is reused, great care should be taken in removing the mask without touching its surfaces and thus contaminating it. Careful fitting is required. Mask testing is done by spraying saccharine on its surface; if one can inhale and taste the saccharine, the mask doesn't meet standards. If one can smell the onions, garlic, or alcohol on someone's breath, he/she are too close, six feet or not.

Current evidence suggests that it is harder to transmit the COVID-19 via a soft surface such as fabric masks or cloth (survives up to 24 hours) than on hard surfaces such as doorknobs, elevator buttons, table tops, silverware, drinking glasses, etc were it can survive for 3-4 days. However, fabric masks and cloth can be laundered in hot water from someone with COVID-19 along with that of the rest of the family, as the temperature is high enough to destroy the virus.

Watch a video explaining the way N95 mask works
https://www.youtube.com/watch?v=eAdanPfQdCA

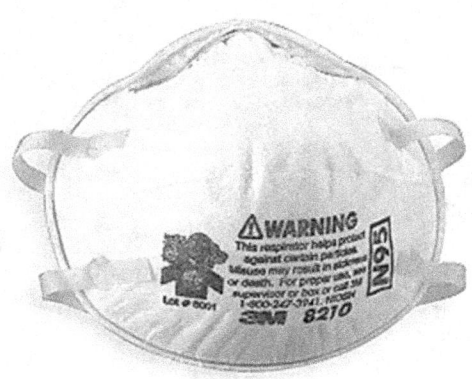

Picture 8: N95 respirator

Beard or facial hair interfere with face mask's efficacy against COVID-19

The CDC recommends wearing face covering (e.g., surgical mask, respirator) in public settings where other social distancing measures are difficult to maintain (e.g., grocery stores, pharmacies), especially in areas of significant community-based transmission. Although neck breathers (laryngectomee and those with tracheostomy) breathe through their stoma, it is recommended that they wear a facemask in addition to covering their stoma with a modified mask or HME.

Ensuring the face mask seal is a vital part of respiratory protection practices. Facial hair that lies along the sealing area of a respirator or face mask, such as beards, sideburns, or some mustaches, will interfere with respirators that rely on a tight face piece seal to achieve maximum protection. (**Picture 9**) Gases, vapors, and virus particles in the air will take the path of least resistance and bypass the part of the respirator that captures or filters hazards out. This can allow the COVID-19 virus access to the respiratory tract.

It is therefore recommended that all individuals including neck breathers remove their facial hair prior to wearing a mask. Shaving may be challenging for those who had radical neck dissection because of their facial numbness. Using an electrical shavers allows safe removal of the hair without injuring the skin.

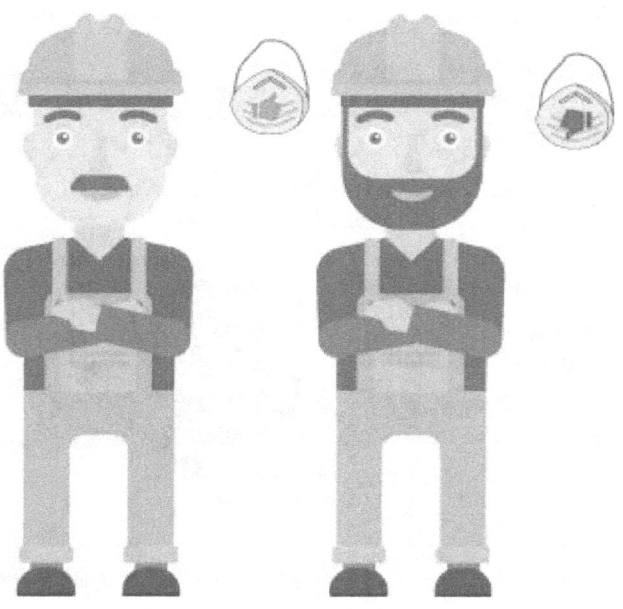

Picture 9: Facial hair and a surgical mask

Protecting immunocompromised patients from COVID-19

Older adults, people who have severe underlying medical conditions such as heart or lung disease or diabetes, and immunocompromised individuals, seem to be at higher risk for developing serious complications from COVID-19 illness. The greater number of risk factors the higher the risk.

Examples of persons with weakened immune systems include those with HIV/AIDS, cancer and transplant patients who are taking certain immunosuppressive drugs, and those with inherited diseases that affect the immune system.

Individuals with cancer including those with head and neck who are at higher risk of suffering from a serious and life threatening COVID -19 infection when they also have the following conditions:

- Age > 55 years

- Pre-existing pulmonary disease

- Chronic kidney and or kidney disease

- Hypertension and/or cardiovascular disease

- Diabetes

- Immunosuppression to include: chronic prednisone treatment (>20 mg/day), biologics, transplant, chemotherapy, and HIV. The risk of developing severe disease may depend on the degree of immune suppression.

These persons as well as those who are in close contact with them should be extra vigilant in following the CDC and local government instructions. It is recommended that they isolating themselves by staying home and avoiding any contact. https://www.cdc.gov/coronavirus/2019-ncov/index.html

It is advisable to contact one's physicians for guidance and when becoming ill.

Coping with COVID-19 pandemic as head and neck cancer patient

The global COVID-19 pandemic is particularly stressful for those undergoing treatment for head and neck cancer, their caretakers, and cancer survivors.

Because of the increasing numbers of patients with COVID-19 infections, many health systems adopted strategies to provide sound care for non COVID-19 patients while reducing the risk of infection transmission to patients and medical personal. Additional considerations include the limited availability of operating rooms and inpatient beds, and the scarcity of personal protective equipment needed to provide safe and hygienic conditions.

Below is a brief outline of some of the changes in the near future prepared by the Head and Neck Cancer Alliance (modified).

People undergoing active treatment (especially chemotherapy) are at increased risk of getting an infection. It is very important that they and those in close contact with them follow the CDC and local government instruction:

- Washing hands with soap and water frequently, for 20 seconds, including wrists.

- If unable to wash hands, using hand sanitizer and rubbing them for 20 seconds.

- Disinfecting commonly used surfaces such as tabletops, doorknobs, and phones.

- Avoiding direct contact with others such as hugging or shaking hands, and staying at least 6 feet away from other people.

- Avoiding being in large groups of six or more people, especially when in an enclosed space.

- Avoiding sharing cups or utensils with others.

- Covering the mouth or stoma during a cough or sneeze.

- Wearing a face mask and protective glasses when at risk of exposure to the virus.

- Avoiding contact with anyone with a known COVID-19 infection or individuals with a cough and/or fever.

- Avoiding air travel or other public transportation.

- Notifying their doctor immediately when feeling sick (develop a cough, fever, muscle aches, or other symptoms) or if after having contact with anyone with a known or suspected COVID-19 infection. It may be necessary to be evaluated and potentially tested for the virus.

Patients who have finished therapy are seen regularly to monitor for cancer recurrence and also to address any of their treatments side effects. In the current crisis, these visits may not be urgent and may increase the risk of exposure to COVID-19 to both survivors and physicians. As a result, many hospitals are postponing non-urgent surgeries, routine follow-up visits and imaging tests (such as CT and PET/CT scans) to minimize the risk of transmission and to conserve health care resources that may be in limited supply. However, if a patient experiences concerning new signs or symptoms for cancer (e.g., worsening mouth or throat pain, changes in one's voice or swallowing, a spot in the mouth that has not healed in 2 weeks, unexplained ear pain, new lump in your neck) he/she should inform their doctor as they may still need to be seen.

A model created by the National Cancer Institute predicts that tens of thousands of excess cancer deaths will occur over the next decade as a result of missed screening, delays in diagnosis, and reductions in oncology treatment caused by the COVID-19 pandemic. It is important that patients continue to be screened and treated.

While social distancing, isolation, and quarantine at home are effective in reducing the incidence of COVID-19, they do increase health risks from other causes. Social isolation among older adults is associated with heightened risk of cardiovascular, autoimmune, neurocognitive, and mental health problems. It is therefore important that individuals do not neglect their medical problems during the pandemic.

Some institutions are offering virtual clinic visits (Telemedicine) interactions with medical providers by way of a video conference call) in an effort to reduce exposure of both patients and health care staff. While virtual visits and telemedicine will never completely replace in-person interactions, in times of crisis, they can provide an effective means to maintain a patient-doctor relationship, allowing them to engage in a directed conversation about disease-specific symptoms and concerns, and to discuss future plans of care. Virtual visits can be very important for head and neck cancer survivors, as they reduce individual patient exposure in clinics and hospitals, and minimize the risk to other cancer patients with compromised immune systems, as well as health care providers and staff. Survivors and caregivers should be reassured that these encounters are a sound approach to cancer surveillance and can allow providers to identify patients who may require an in-person visit.

Other general considerations:

- Maintaining close communication with family/loved ones and health care team

- Having a sufficient supply (at least a 2-week supply) of easy to preserve food items, prescriptions and cleaning supplies and other essentials.

- Contacting one's physician to ensure one has adequate access to prescription medications, and necessary supplies (e.g., tube feedings, tracheostomy supplies and personal protective equipment)

Neck breathers (laryngectomees and those with tracheostomy) are likely at higher risk of becoming infected with COVID-19 due to the increased exposure of their airway. These individuals should observe special precautions (See above).

COVID-19 testing in laryngectomees

Two kinds of tests are available for COVID-19: viral tests and antibody tests.

- A viral test tells if someone has a current infection. It is obtained by collecting a nasopharyngeal specimen (e.g., nasal, oropharyngeal) with a swab. Neck breathers should be tested in two locations: by collecting a nasopharyngeal specimen as well as a stomal specimen. See the American Academy of Otolaryngology recommendations https://www.ahns.info/wp-content/uploads/2020/04/Policy-for-COVID-testing-of-patients-with-stomas-4.7.2020.pdf .
- An antibody test is obtained by getting a blood sample. It tells if a person had a previous infection.

Those whose viral test is positive and are sick or take care of someone need to take protective steps.

A negative viral test result only means that the person tested did not have COVID-19 at the time of testing. If the viral test is positive or negative for COVID-19, the person tested still should take preventive measures to protect themselves and others.

An antibody test may not be able to show if a person has a current infection, because it can take 1-3 weeks after infection to make antibodies. Currently it is not know if having antibodies to the virus can protect someone from getting infected with the virus again, or how long that protection might last.

An article by Sethuraman et al. (https://jamanetwork.com/journals/jama/fullarticle/2765837) describes how to interpret 2 types of diagnostic tests commonly in use for SARS-CoV-2 infections—reverse transcriptase–polymerase chain reaction (RT-PCR) and IgM and IgG enzyme-linked immunosorbent assay (ELISA)—and how the results may vary over time.

CDC has guidance for who should be tested, but decisions about testing are made by state and local health departments or healthcare providers.

See more details at https://www.cdc.gov/coronavirus/2019-ncov/symptoms-testing/testing.html and https://www.cdc.gov/coronavirus/2019-nCoV/lab/index.html

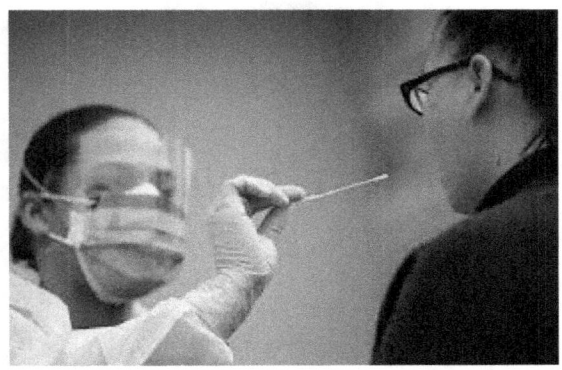

Picture 10: Obtaining a swab specimen

Chapter 2:

Psychological and social issues in head and neck patients (including laryngectomees) caused by the COVID-19 pandemic

---

Mental health issues in head and neck patients (including laryngectomees) caused by the COVID-19 pandemic

The current COVID-19 outbreak is spurring depression, fear, anxiety, and stress on a societal level. An increase in deaths by suicide during this quarantine period was also noted. On an individual level, it may exacerbate anxiety and psychosis-like symptoms as well as lead to non-specific mental issues (e.g., mood problems, sleep issues, phobia-like behaviors, panic-like symptoms). Head and neck cancer patients (HNCP) are more vulnerable to these psychological issues as well as the viral infection. Laryngectomees may experience increased social isolation and loneliness.

Contributing to these are the difficulties in get medical and diagnostic care, prescription drugs, and medical supplies, and the economic situation.

HNCP with mental health issues such as obsessive-compulsive disorders (OCD) and post-traumatic stress disorder (PTSD), anxiety and depressive disorders, and paranoia may experience exacerbation of their symptoms.

HNCP can be proactive and alleviate some of their psychological vulnerability by:

- Reaching out and seeking support from mental health professionals (e.g., psychiatrists, psychologists, social workers)

- Getting medical and other supplies delivered to one's residence

- Engaging in healthy distractions such as reading, watching movies, taking walks, exercising, and learning a new skill

- Developing a routine

- Obtaining information from reliable sources
- Curbing media exposure to certain times in the day

- Being aware of what is anxiety and what is reality in one's thoughts and conversations

- Following guidelines (i.e., using prescribed handwashing methods, avoiding touching the face, avoiding hugging and shaking hands, staying at home and contacting one's medical provider when experiencing medical problems)

- Connecting with family and friends through the internet, social media, video calls and phone

Following these guidelines can assist HNCP navigate through the corona virus pandemic.

Coping with depression

Many individuals feel depressed as a result of the COVID-19 pandemic. The social isolation, fear of becoming infected, and difficulties in getting medical and dental care contribute to this feeling. Laryngectomees are more prone to feel depressed because of their difficulty to communicate and their daily struggle to deal with their handicaps and limitations. Yet the social stigma associated with admitting depression makes it difficult to reach out and seek therapy.

Some of the signs of depression include:

- A feeling of helplessness and hopelessness, or that life has no meaning

- No interest in being with family or friends

- Inability to communicate

- Difficulty paying attention

- No interest in the hobbies and activities one used to enjoy

- A loss of appetite, or no interest in food

- Crying for long periods of time, or many times each day

- Sleep problems, either sleeping too much or too little

- Changes in energy level and apathy

- Wide mood swings raging from elation to despair

- Feeling isolated

- Changes in sexual desire

- Thoughts of suicide, including making plans or taking action to kill oneself, as well as frequently thinking about death and dying

The challenges of life as a laryngectomee in the shadow of cancer means that it is even more difficult to deal with depression. Being unable to speak, or even having difficulties with speaking, make it harder to express emotions and can lead to isolation. Surgical and medical care is often not sufficient to address such issues; more emphasis should be given to mental well-being after laryngectomy.

Coping with and overcoming depression are very important, not only for the well-being of the patient, but also to facilitate recovery, and increase one's chance for survival and ultimate cure. There is growing scientific evidence of a connection between mind and body. Although many of these connections are not yet understood, it is well recognized that individuals who are motivated to get better and exhibit a positive attitude recover faster from serious illnesses, live longer and sometimes survive immense odds.

Individuals who experience suicidal thoughts are encourage to seek help from mental health professionals such as social workers, psychologist and psychiatrist. They can call the National Suicide Prevention Lifeline at 1-800-273-8255 to get immediate assistance.

Overcoming depression

Hopefully one can find the strength within to fight depression especially during the COVID-pandemic.

Some of the ways laryngectomee and head and neck cancer patients can overcome depression include:

- Avoid substance abuse

- Seek help from your doctor, nurse, or a member of your health care team with whom you feel comfortable

- Exclude medical causes (e.g., hypothyroidism, side effect of medication)

- Determine to become proactive

- Minimize stress

- Set an example for others

- Return to previous activities

- Talk to a psychologist or social worker

- Consider antidepressant medication

- Seek support from family, friends, professional, colleagues, fellow laryngectomees, and support groups

These are some of the ways of renewing one's spirit:

- Develop leisure activities

- Build personal relationships

- Keep physically fit and active

- Social reintegration with family and friends
- Volunteer

- Find purposeful projects

- Rest

Support by family members and friends is very important. Continuous involvement and contribution to others lives can be invigorating. One can draw strength from enjoying, interacting and influencing the lives of their children and grandchildren. Setting an example to one's children and grandchildren not to give up in the face of adversity can be the driving force to be proactive and resist depression.

Getting involved in activities one liked before the surgery can provider a continuous purpose for life. Participating in the activities of a local laryngectomee club can be a new source of support, advice and friendship.

Seeking the help of a mental health professional such as a social worker, psychologist or psychiatrist can also be very helpful. This may be more difficult during the pandemic and utilizing telemedicine can be helpful. There are many treatment options for depression. These include psychotherapy, medications, and transcranial magnetic stimulation. Having a caring and competent physician and a speech and language pathologist who can provide continuous follow-up is very important. Their involvement can help patients deal with emerging medical and speech problems and can contribute to their sense of well-being.

Individuals who experience suicidal thoughts are encourage to seek help from mental health professionals such as social workers, psychologist and psychiatrist. They can call the National Suicide Prevention Lifeline at 1-800-273-8255 to get immediate assistance.

How laryngectomees can cope with the COVID -19 quarantine

The forced quarantine imposed by COVID -19 can be difficult for laryngectomees. Their communication difficulties may increase their social isolation, leading to medical and psychological problems.

In addition to taking steps to improve psychological vulnerability (e.g., developing a routine, reading, watching movies, taking walks, exercising, and learning a new skill),

Laryngectomees may want to consider the following:

- Communicating with family, friends and support groups by speaking over the phone; and e-mailing and texting using computer, tablet and smartphone. There are several applications that allow video communication (e.g., Skype, FaceTime, Zoom) to keep in touch. The volume and quality of the voice when using telecommunication methods can be improved by using a hand held microphone and placing it near the laptop, iPad or iPhone (**Picture 11**) It would be helpful for support groups to continue meeting using some of these methods.

- Those using tracheo-esophageal speech can learn how to communicate through other methods of speaking (e.g., esophageal speech, electrolarynx, sign language) in case they need to plug their leaking voice prosthesis.

- Not ignoring medical, dental and psychological issues. Continuing to receive care from physicians, dentists, mental health providers, and speech and language pathologists. If physical access to them is limited, contacting them using telemedicine.

- Having adequate supplies needed to speak and care for the airways (e.g., baseplate, HME, saline bullets).

As home confinement and other restrictions are being lifted, it would be prudent for laryngectomees to continue to observe precautionary measures. As more clinical experience in managing COVID-19 infection is gained and new medications and vaccines are available the consequences of becoming infected may become less dangerous.

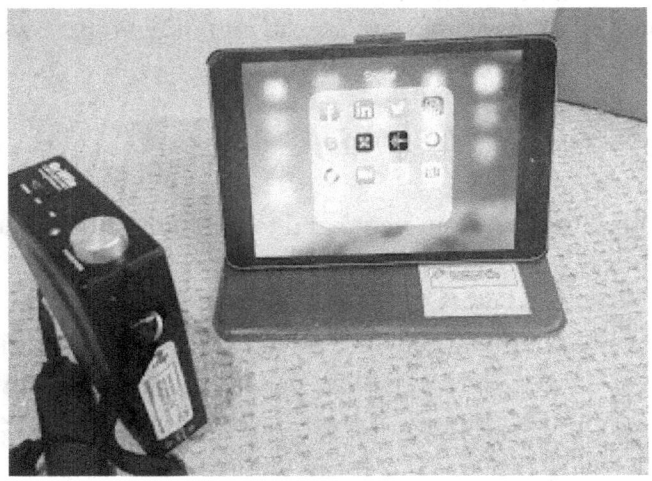

Picture 11: Placing the voice amplifier near the iPad increases voice volume

Going outside during the COVID-19 pandemic. What should laryngectomees do?

Laryngectomee may experience social and medical challenges when they leave their home during the COVID-19 pandemics. Most non-neck breathers do not understand or recognize their medical condition and may react in a negative way toward them. They may be alarmed when the laryngectomee coughs or sneezes, or take care of their stoma in public.

Some of the steps that laryngectomees can take when in public are:

- Cleaning the stoma and trachea including inserting saline into the trachea and coughing out the secretions before going out

- Taking care of the stoma and it's secretions at a private location away from others (e.g., bathroom, separate room)

- Covering the stoma (with napkin, cloth or elbow) whenever coughing or sneezing. Preferably, this is done away from other people. When coughing forcefully the stoma can produce a large amount of droplets that can spread and infect others when the laryngectomee carries a respiratory virus such as COVID-19

- Keeping a distance of at least 6 feet (2 meters) from others

- A useful routine is to use the non-dominant hand to touch the stoma and the dominant hand for other activities (e.g., touching a door handle).

- Wearing a surgical mask or garment over the mouth and nose (in addition another one over the stoma). This is done to protect the laryngectomee from becoming infected, as well as others when the laryngectomee is infected. Wearing a mask over the mouth and nose in public prevent the laryngectomee from standing out from others. Wearing the mask on the stoma and face also serves in preventing laryngectomees from touching these locations with unclean hands.

As home confinement and other restrictions are being slowly lifted, it would be prudent for laryngectomees to continue to observe these precautionary measures. As more clinical experience in managing COVID-19 infection is gained and new medications and vaccines are available the consequences of becoming infected may become less dangerous.

How to avoid and cope with quarantine fatigue

Months into the COVID-19 pandemic, the effects of the disease and public safety precautions have been devastating — mental health and addiction issues have risen, jobs have been lost and, tragically, tens of thousands have lost their lives. Some have simply become weary of the monotony and loneliness of staying at home. These lonely and isolation can be more severe in laryngectomees and head and neck cancer survivors who have communication difficulties.

All of this has led to what experts are calling "COVID-19 quarantine fatigue," a modern-day version of what is known as "caution fatigue." This is a phenomenon when one's body and mind tire of the persistent sense of danger and the constant stress it is causing, leading to becoming complacent or unable to make good decisions.

What is COVID-19 quarantine fatigue?

With quarantine fatigue, one might grow weary of — or actively ignore — the precautions that can slow the spread of COVID-19. The sense of urgency in managing the global health emergency may fade, leading to impatient or tiredness of complying with the health and safety guidelines.

One may begin to feel hopeless, as if no amount of measures can keep one safe from exposure. This can result in decreasing the home sanitizing and forgetting to wear a face covering when going out. Some may expand the number of people they spend time with in person or forego all precautionary measures.

There is an understandable eagerness to 'go back to normal.' Since the virus is invisible, it may seem that it does not really exist, even though there is evidence it is still spreading. There is a genuine desire to and interact and connect with others and deny or ignore the health risks associated with the virus.

It is important to resist quarantine fatigue and remember that we are all in this together and it takes cooperation from everyone in the community to decrease the spread of COVID-19. Yielding to isolation fatigue can cause an increase in COVID-19 cases as well as repeated lockdowns and further shuttering of businesses and schools. A rise in infection rates, can overwhelm the health care system, and increased deaths in those who are vulnerable.

Resisting quarantine fatigue is especially important in older adults, people who have severe underlying medical conditions and immunocompromised individuals who are at higher risk for developing serious complications from COVID-19 illness.

How to cope with quarantine fatigue:

Enclosed are recommendations how to avoid quarantine fatigue and continue being diligent in the collective efforts to keep our community healthy and reduce the number of COVID-19 infections:

- Staying informed with trusted and reliable resources, such as the Centers for Disease Control and Prevention (CDC) website.
- Avoiding constant exposure to news, though it may be beneficial to check local news at occasional intervals to learn pertinent details about COVID-19 in your community.
- Taking care of oneself — eating a nutritionally balanced diet, exercising, getting appropriate amounts of sleep, practicing self-care, and taking care of one's medical needs.
- Staying connected with loved ones, friend and support groups.
- Maintaining precautions to avoid catching or spreading the disease.

Chapter 3:

How to take care of voice prosthesis leakage or dislodgement during the corona pandemic

---

Coping with voice prosthesis leakage or dislodgement during the corona (COVID- 19) pandemic

The corona (COVID-19) pandemic presents many challenges for laryngectomees and their medical providers. Because of the reduction or decrease in outpatient services and voice prosthesis availability, those using tracheoesophageal speech may have trouble in having their clinician-changed (indwelling) prosthesis replaced because of leakage through or around the prosthesis. A patient with a leak around or through the voice prosthesis is at an increased risk of aspiration with potential sequelae including pneumonia, which could lead to devastating outcomes if patients contract COVID-19.

Enclosed are suggestions how to cope with these challenges:

- If possible, switching to using patient-changed voice prosthesis (non indwelling)

- Extending the life span of the current voice prosthesis by keeping it clean using a cleaning brush and flushing bulb and preventing buildup of candida biofilm (see below).

If voice prosthesis leakage occurs:

- Attempting to stop the leak by cleaning and brushing it as suggested in The Laryngectomee Guide (pages 75-19) or at http://dribrook.blogspot.com/p/tracheo-esophageal-voice-prosthesis-tep.html

- Stopping the leak by inserting an adequate plug (**Picture 12**) into the prosthesis whenever consuming fluids or leaving it permanently and switching to alternate speaking method (e.g., esophageal speech, electrolarynx)

- Consuming viscous fluids that generally do not leak (e.g., yogurt, jelly, soup, oatmeal, etc) through or around the prosthesis

- Drinking small amount of fluid without strong effort while lying down, swallowing the liquid as if it is a food item, speaking a few words each time fluids are swallowed, can reduce or prevent the liquids from leaking into the trachea

- If the prosthesis has been accidentally removed or dislodged (not aspirated), a 12 Fr/16''red rubber catheter (**Picture 13**) or puncture dilator can be inserted into the trachea-esophageal puncture to prevent its closure until the voice prosthesis is replaced. An advantage to using a rubber catheter is that the red rubber catheter can serve as alternate means of nutrition until prosthesis replacement becomes is possible.

The laryngectomee should seek immediate medical care if aspiration of the dislodged voice prosthesis has occurred as this may requires urgent intervention to remove it.

It is helpful to contact one's speech and language pathologist and/or physician for guidance and when voice prosthesis leakage occurs.

More information how to prevent and deal with voice prosthesis leakage can be found in the sections below. Information is also available in The Laryngectomee Guide http://goo.gl/z8RxEt and My Voice website at http://dribrook.blogspot.com/p/tracheo-esophageal-voice-prosthesis-tep.html

Watch a video that explains what to do if the voice prosthesis leaks at:
Https://www.youtube.com/watch?v=w0K98HtE308&feature=youtu.be

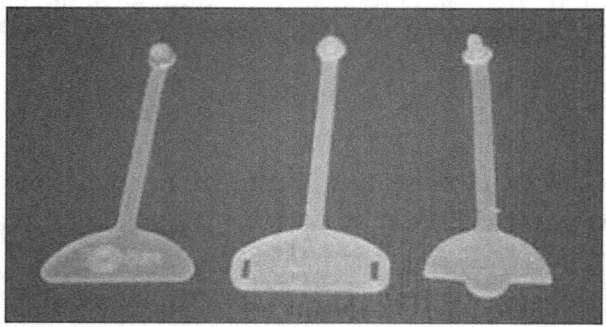

Picture 12: Voice prosthesis plugs

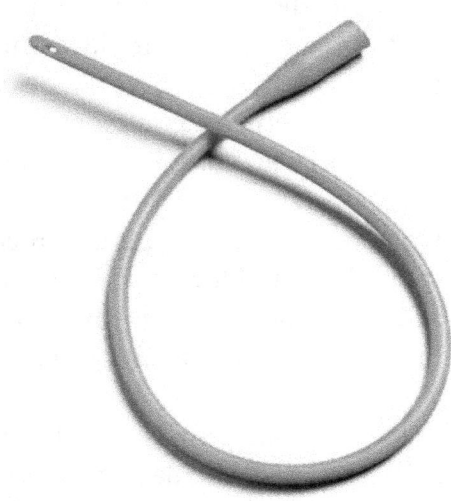

Picture 13: Red Catheter

Cleaning the voice prosthesis and preventing leaking

It is very important to keep the voice prosthesis clean to insure its proper function and durability. When not cleaned properly the prosthesis can leak, and the ability to speak can be compromised or weakened. It is recommended that the inner space (lumen) of the voice prosthesis be cleaned at least twice a day (morning and evening), and preferably after eating because this is the time when food and mucus can become trapped. Sometimes mucus blocks the prosthesis (when getting up in the morning or after eating) which interfere with the ability to speak. Cleaning is especially helpful after eating sticky foods or whenever one's voice is weak.

A prosthesis cleaning brush and flushing bulb are used in cleaning the prosthesis.

Maintenance and prevention of leakage

Maintenance and prevention of leakage guidelines are:

- Before using the brush provided by the manufacturer (**Picture 14**), dip it in a cup of hot water and leave it there for a few seconds.

- Initially the mucus around the prosthesis should be cleaned using tweezers preferably with rounded tips. Following that, the manufacturer-provided brush should be inserted into the prosthesis (not too deep) and twisted around a few times back and forth. The brush should be thoroughly washed with warm water after each cleaning. The prosthesis is then flushed twice with warm (not hot) water using the manufacturer's provided bulb.

- Take the brush out and rinse it with hot water and repeat the process 2-3 times until no material is brought out by the brush. Wait until the brush is not hot any more before brushing the prosthesis again. Be careful not to insert it beyond the voice prosthesis inner valve to avoid traumatizing the esophagus with excessive heat.

- Flush the voice prosthesis twice using the bulb provided by the manufacturer(**Picture 15**) using warm (not hot!) potable water. To avoid damage to the esophagus sip the water first to make sure that the water temperature is not too high.The flushing bulb should be introduced into the prosthesis opening while applying slight pressure to completely seal off the opening. The angle that one should place the tip of the bulb varies between individuals. (The SLP can provide instructions how to choose the best angle.) Flushing the prosthesis should be done gently because using too much pressure can lead to splashing of water into the trachea. If flushing with water is problematic, the flush can also be used with air

- Prevent formation of biofilm by yeast and bacteria (see below)

Warm water works better than room temperature water in cleansing the prosthesis probably because it dissolves the dry secretions and mucus and perhaps even flushes away (or even kills) some of the yeast colonies that had formed on the prosthesis.

The manufacturers of each voice prosthesis brush and flushing bulb provide directions of how to clean them and when they should be discarded. The brush should be replaced when its threads become bent or worn out.

The prosthesis brush and flushing bulb should be cleaned with hot water, when possible, and soap and dried with a towel after every use. One way to keep them clean is to place them on a clean towel and expose them to sunlight for a few hours, on a daily basis. This takes advantage of the antibacterial power of the sun's ultraviolet light to reduce the number of bacteria and fungi.

Placing 2-3 cc of sterile saline (**Picture 16**) in the trachea at least twice a day (and more if the air is dry), wearing an HME 24/7 and using a humidifier can keep the mucus moist and reduce the clogging of the voice prosthesis.

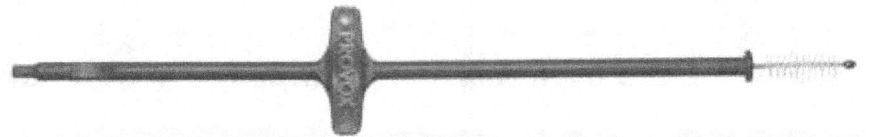

Picture 14: A voice prosthesis cleaning brush (Atos Medical)

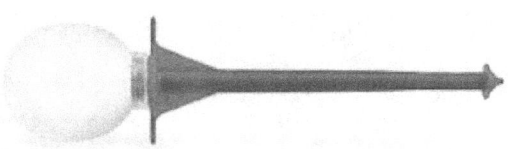

Picture 15: A voice prosthesis flushing bulb (Atos Medical)

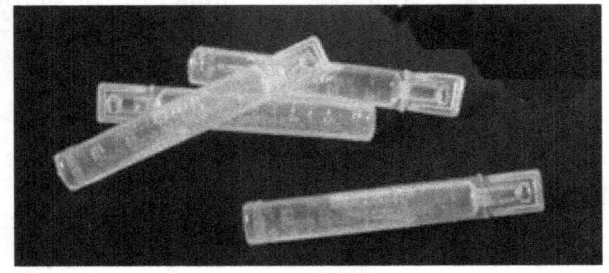

Picture 16: A sterile saline vial for respiratory tract use ("Saline bullet")

Preventing biofilm of yeast and bacteria from growing on the voice prosthesis

Overgrowth of yeast and bacteria in the form of a biofilm (a thin, slimy film of microorganisms that adheres to a surface) on the voice prosthesis is one cause of the prosthesis leaking and thus failing. Nevertheless, it takes some time for yeast and bacteria to grow in a newly installed voice prosthesis and form the biofilm that prevent its valve's from closing completely. Accordingly, failures immediately after voice prosthesis installation are unlikely due to yeast growth. Formulation of biofilm on the valve may also lead to increased air flow resistance making it harder to speak.

The presence of yeast should be established by the person who changes the failing voice prosthesis This can be done by observing the typical yeast (Candida) colonies that prevent the valve from closing and, if possible, by sending a specimen from the voice prosthesis for fungal culture.

The antifungal agents Mycostatin and Clotrimazole (Mycelex) troches, can be used to prevent voice prosthesis failure due to yeast. They are available with a prescription in the form of a suspension or tablets (Mycostain) and troches (Mycelex). Mycostatin tablets can be crushed and dissolved in water. There is anecdotal information that apple cider vinegar that is known to inhibit candida growth can be used to gargle and be swallowed to prevent yeast growth on the voice prosthesis.

Automatically administering anti-fungal therapy (e.g., mycostatin) just because one assumes that yeast is the cause of voice prosthesis failure may be inappropriate without proof. It is expensive, may lead to the yeast developing resistance to the agent, and may cause unnecessary side effects.

There are, however, exceptions to this rule. These include the administration of preventive anti-fungal agents to diabetics; those receiving antibiotics; chemotherapy or steroid; and those where colonization with yeast is evident (coated tongue etc.).

There are several methods that help prevent yeast from growing on the voice prosthesis:

- Reduce the consumption of sugars in food and drinks, brush your teeth well after consuming sugary food and/or drinks.

- Brush your teeth well after every meal and especially before going to sleep.

- Clean your dentures daily.

- Diabetic should maintain adequate blood sugar levels.

- Take antibiotics and corticosteroids only if they are needed.

- After using an oral suspension of an antifungal agent, wait for 30 minutes to let it work and then brush your teeth. This is because some of these suspensions contain sugar.

- Dip the voice prosthesis brush in a small amount of mycostatin suspension or vinegar and brush the inner voice prosthesis before going to sleep. (A homemade suspension can be made by dissolving a quarter of a mycostatin tablet in 3-5 cc water). This would leave some of the suspension inside the voice prosthesis. The unused suspension should be discarded. Do not place too much mycostatin or vinegar in the prosthesis to prevent dripping into the trachea. Speaking a few words after placing the suspension will push it towards the inner part of the voice prosthesis.

- Consume probiotics by eating active-culture yogurt and/or a probiotic preparation.

- Gently brush the tongue if it is coated with yeast (white plaques)

- Replace the toothbrush after overcoming a yeast problem to prevent re colonizing with yeasts

- Keep the prosthesis brush clean

Chapter 4:

Mucus, respiratory care, and fitness during the COVID-19 pandemic

---

Mucus production and increasing air humidity

Prior to becoming a laryngectomee, the inhaled air is warmed to body temperature, humidified and cleansed of organisms and dust particles by the filtration capacity of the upper part of the respiratory system. Since these functions do not occur following laryngectomy, it is important to restore the lost functions previously provided by the upper part of the respiratory system. These practices should be continued during the COVID-19 pandemic.

When the inhaled air humidity is too low the trachea can dry out, crack, and produce some bleeding. If the bleeding is significant or does not respond to an increase in humidity, a physician should be consulted. In addition, if the amount or color of the mucus is concerning, one should contact their physician.

Tracheal dryness, irritation and overproduction of mucus can lead to the development of mucus plugs. These plugs can cause airway obstruction that can lead to collapse of sections (atelectasis) of the lungs. An irritated trachea may be more susceptible to COVID-19 and other respiratory tract viruses.

Steps to achieve better humidification and healthier mucus production include:

- Wearing an heat and moisture exchanger (HME) filter 24/7 which keeps the tracheal moisture higher and preserves the heat inside the trachea and lungs

- Wetting the soma cover (or bib) to breathe moist air (in those who wear a stoma cover). Although less effective than an HME, dampening the foam filter or stoma cover with clean plain water can also assist in increasing humidification.

- Drinking enough fluid to keep well hydrated

- Inserting 3-5 cc saline (preferably using saline "Bullets") into the stoma 3 to 5 times a day

- Using a humidifier in the house to achieve about 40-50% humidity and getting a hygrometer to monitor the humidity. This is important both in the summer when air conditioning is used, and in the winter when heating is used

- Using nebulizing bottle twice daily

- Breathing steam generated by boiling water or a hot shower

.

More information about treatment of these conditions can be obtained in The Laryngectomee Guide at http://bit.ly/38BJUnt and https://dribrook.blogspot.com/p/mucous-and-airway-care.html

Respiratory rehabilitation

After laryngectomy the inhaled air bypasses the upper part of the respiratory system and enters the trachea and lungs directly through the stoma. The change effects the efforts needed to breathe and potential lung functions. This requires adjustment and retraining. Breathing is actually easier for laryngectomees because there is less airflow resistance when the air bypasses the nose and mouth. Because it is easier to get air into the lungs, laryngectomees no longer need to inflate and deflate their lungs as completely as they did before. It is therefore common for laryngectomees to develop reduced lung capacity and breathing capabilities. This may eventually lead to collapse of portions of the base of the lower lobs of the lungs (atelectasis). Atelectasis of portions of the lungs may increase the risk of acquiring respiratory virus infections and make it more difficult to adequately ventilate the patient.

There are several measures available to laryngectomees that can preserve and increase their lung capacity:

- The use of a heat and moisture exchanger filter (HME) can create resistance to air exchange. This forces the individual to fully inflate their lungs to get the needed amount of oxygen.

- Regular breathing exercises under medical supervision and guidance of a respiratory therapist. This can get the lungs to fully inflate and improve individuals' heart and breathing capacities. One way to improve breathing capacity is by using a modified incentive spirometer (a device that make the ball rise to the indicated range). One can mark their progress with a siding pointer. (**Picture 17**) The spirometer can be modified for laryngectomee use by replacing the mouthpiece with a large diameter baby bottle nipple that fits over stoma. Another way to expand the lungs is to take 2 to 3 deep breaths, hold, and slowly let the air out.

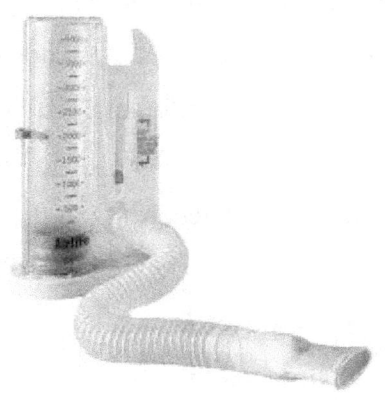

Picture 17: Incentive spirometer

- Using diaphragmatic breathing. This method of breathing allows for greater utilization of the lung capacity. This can breathing method can be used when resting or exercising (e.g., walking, biking). (see below)

More information about treatment of these conditions can be obtained in The Laryngectomee Guide at http://bit.ly/38BJUnt   and https://dribrook.blogspot.com/p/mucous-and-airway-care.html

Keeping fit and eating adequate nutrition during the COVID-19 pandemic

Keeping fit and exercising during the COVID-19 pandemic can be difficult. As people self-isolate and practice social distancing, many gyms are closed. At the same time, it is important than that laryngectomees keep exercising and staying as active as possible – for both their mental and physical health. Performing fitness exercises and riding stationary bikes can be done at home and provide an excellent mode of keeping fit. Taking walks outside while keeping social distancing and wearing protective mask and HME is helpful.

People who eat a well-balanced diet tend to be healthier with stronger immune systems and have a lower risk of chronic illnesses and infectious diseases. Eating adequate diet is very important and may be challenging for laryngectomees with swallowing difficulties. (see more at https://dribrook.blogspot.com/p/eating-and-swallowing-issues.html .) Proper nutrition and hydration during the COVID-19 outbreak are vital according to the World Health Organization (WHO) (http://www.emro.who.int/nutrition/nutrition-infocus/nutrition-advice-for-adults-during-the-covid-19-outbreak.html) Their nutrition advice for adults is to eat a variety of fresh and unprocessed foods every day to get the vitamins, minerals, dietary fiber, protein and antioxidants the body needs. Drinking enough water is also important. The WHO recommends avoiding sugar, fat and salt to significantly lower the risk of overweight, obesity, heart disease, stroke, diabetes and certain types of cancer.

Chapter 5:

Treating fibrosis and lymphedema and dealing with esophageal dilation

---

Fibrosis and lymphedema treatment during the COVID-19 pandemic

It is important that individuals who received radiation treatment and/or surgery for head and neck cancer continue treating their post radiation neck and face fibrosis and lymphadenitis.

This may be difficult during the COVID-19 pandemic as access the physical therapists and lymphedema specialist may be limited or absent. Some therapists offer treatment using telemedicine. Most therapist encourage their patients to continue using their treatment modalities and exercises at home.

Treatment of **fibrosis** that can be done at home and includes stretching the neck muscles by exercises such as chin curls, head rotations, shoulder shrugs, and shoulder circles. Exercise can reduce neck tightness and increases the range of neck motion. One needs to perform these exercises throughout life to maintain good neck mobility.

Treatment of **lymphedema** that can be done at home include manual lymph drainage, compression bandages and garments, remedial exercises, and skin care.

It is best to consult one's therapists to inquire about the appropriate treatment modalities they should follow.

More information about treatment of these conditions can be obtained in The Laryngectomee Guide at http://bit.ly/38BJUnt and https://dribrook.blogspot.com/p/lymphedema-and-neck-swelling.html (for lymphedema) and https://dribrook.blogspot.com/p/radiation-side-effects.html (for fibrosis)

How to cope with neopharyngeal or esophageal narrowing during the COVID-19 pandemic

The corona (COVID-19) pandemic presents many challenges for head and neck cancer patients and their medical providers. Because of the reduction or decrease in outpatient services, the availability of neopharyngeal and /or esophageal dilation for esophageal narrowing may not be available.

Enclosed are suggestions how to cope with these challenges:

- Performing dilation at-home using self-dilation device

- Considering treatment that resolve the narrowing (i.e., stent, laser treatment)

- Temporarily altering the diet to soft or liquid one

- Using a gastric tube for feeding

It is helpful to contact one's speech and language pathologist and/or physician for guidance. Many institutions perform dilation to those who are unable to consume sufficient calories and liquids.

More information about treatment of these conditions can be obtained in The Laryngectomee Guide at http://bit.ly/38BJUnt and https://dribrook.blogspot.com/p/eating-and-swallowing-issues.html

Chapter 6:

Hospitalization

Admission to the hospital requires preparation for laryngectomees because of their special needs in supplies and their difficulties in communication. It is best to prepare for a potential admission beforehand in case it is an urgent one.

Preparing a kit with essential information and material when going to the hospital

It is helpful to have a plan in place in case one becomes sick. Identifying a caregiver and staying in touch with family, friends, neighbors, and healthcare professionals during the pandemic through email or phone, especially if some lives alone is important. If one is aware of an exposure or are experiencing symptoms such as a sore throat, dry cough, fever, and/or shortness of breath, seek medical help as soon as possible. Trying to contact one's care team over the phone before coming into a medical center can facilitate their care.

Laryngectomees may need to receive emergency and non-emergency medical care at a hospital or other medical facility. Because of their difficulty in communicating with medical personnel and providing information, especially when in distress it is helpful to prepare a folder with this information. Additionally it is useful to carry a kit (**Picture 18**) containing items and supplies needed to maintain their ability to communicate and care for their stoma. The kit should be kept in a place that is easily accessible in an emergency.

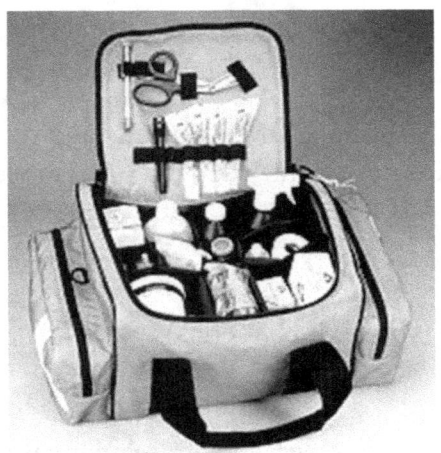

Picture 18: Emergency kit

The kit should contain the following:

- An updated summary of the medical and surgical history, allergies and diagnoses

- An updated list of the medications taken and the results of all procedures, and results of radiological examinations, scans and laboratory tests. These may be placed on a disc or USB flash drive

- Contact information and proof of medical insurance

- Information (phone, email, address) of the laryngectomee's physician(s), speech and language pathologist, family members and friend(s)

- A figure or drawing of a side view of the neck that explains the anatomy of the laryngectomee's upper airways and if relevant where the voice prosthesis is located

- A paper pad and pen

- An electrolarynx with extra batteries (even for those using a voice prosthesis)

- A box of paper tissues

- A supply of saline bullets, HME filters, HME housing, and supplies needed to apply and remove them (e.g., alcohol, Remove, Skin Tag, glue) and to clean the voice prosthesis (brush, flushing bulb)

- Tweezers, mirror, flash light (with extra batteries)

Having these items available when seeking emergency or regular care can be critically important. It is also important to wearing a bracelet or a wristband that identifies the laryngectomee as neck breathers. (**Picture 19**).

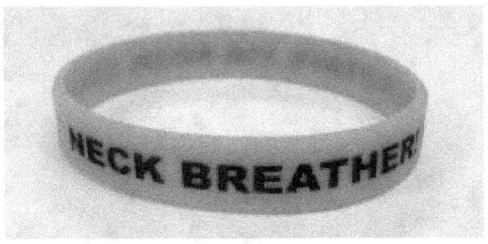

Picture 19: Neck breather's wristband

Ensuring adequate care during hospitalization for neck breathers including laryngectomees

Neck breathers are at a high risk of receiving inadequate care when hospitalized. The medical staff is often not aware of their condition, do not know how to care for their airways, and may not know how to communicate with them.

The COVID-19 pandemic created greater workload for hospital staff and may make it difficult to pay attention to laryngectomee's special needs. Because most hospital limit or prohibit the presence of patients' companions, making it more difficult for laryngectomees to communicate with the staff.

It is therefore important to take certain steps to ensure that the care is adequate:

1. Inform the ward's head nurse and attending physician about the laryngectomee's general and specific needs. In case of elective admission, this can be done prior to the admission to allow the staff time to get ready and to get adequate supplies and equipment.

2. Remind the ward's head nurse, attending physician and anesthetist (when undergoing a procedure with sedation or surgery) about the proper way of administrating anesthesia, suctioning, ventilating and intubation). Show them the video in YouTube: https://goo.gl/Unstch The video is also available in DVD that can be obtained free from Atos medical. (**Picture 20**)

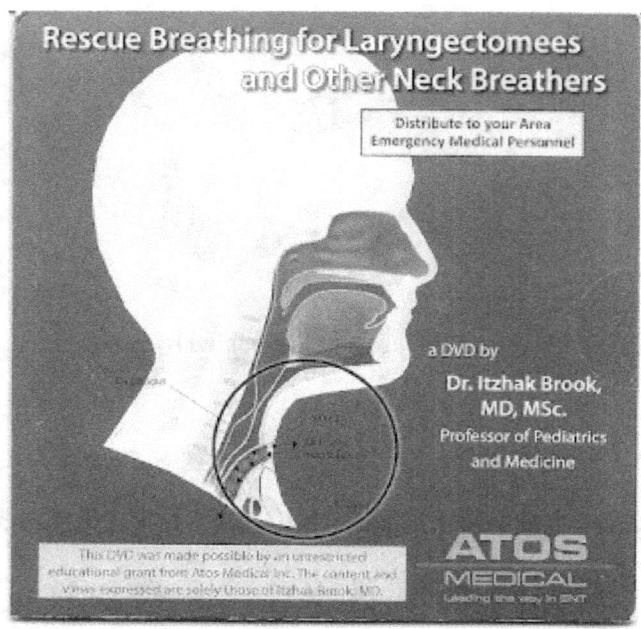

Picture 20: DVD of rescue breathing of laryngectomees

3. Inform the dietitian about the food requirements of the laryngectomee.

4. Inform and, when possible, meet with the hospital's speech and language pathologist to ensure adequate care and availability of adequate supplies.

5. Laryngectomees who experience swallowing difficulties should request that the orally administered medications be given in liquid or easy to swallow form.

6. Request specific supplies and equipment to ensure adequate respiratory care, such as saline bullets, humidifier, and suction machine.

7. Keep reminding every staff member caring for the laryngectomee about his or her condition. This can be done by the patient and/or advocate.

8. Inform the head nurse; attending physician, and/or patient's hospital advocate if medical care is not adequate or if errors are made.

9. Request that signs informing the staff about the laryngectomee be placed in the patient's room. (**Picture 21**)

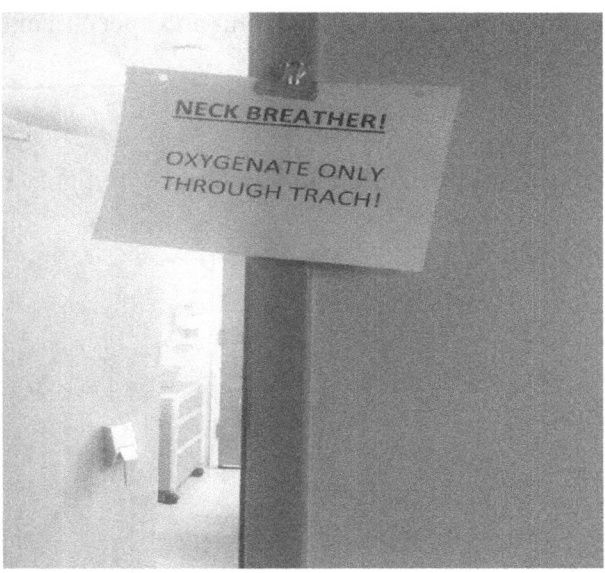

Picture 21: Signs in patient's hospital room informing the staff about the laryngectomee

10. Wear the hospital patient ID wristband on the same hand that identifies them as neck breathers. (**Picture 22**) Because staff is required to continuously check the patient ID wristband, they will be reminded of the condition.

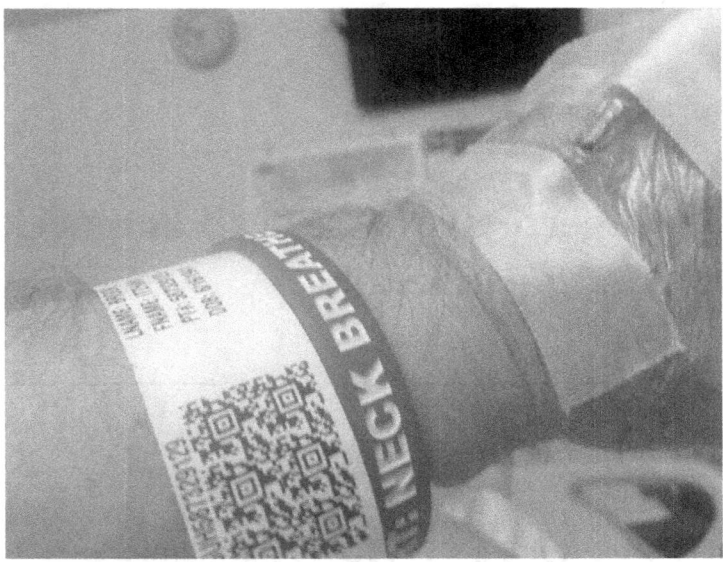

Picture 22: Wearing the hospital patient ID wristband on the same hand

11. Make sure that the laryngectomee is able to communicate with staff. Those using tracheoesophageal speech may need to use alternative speech methods such as an electrolarynx and/or communicate through writing and speech generating devices, i.e., laptop, smartphone, etc.

12. Preparing a kit with essential information and material when going to the hospital (See above)

Chapter 7:

Guidelines for laryngectomees and head and neck cancer care during COVID-19 pandemic

---

Head and neck cancer care during COVID-19 pandemic

Neck breathers (including laryngectomees) infected with COVID-19 carry a high risk of transmitting the virus to other individuals by aerosolizing tracheal secretions to their environment. Infection control strategies specific to patients with laryngectomy should be adhered whenever they are cared for.

Personal protective equipment (PPE) should be adequately utilized, and only necessary medical providers should be in the treatment or patient's room. Patients should always be presumed positive with COVID-19, until proven otherwise. It is recommended that whenever they care for a laryngectomee medical providers wear a N95 respirator and face shield or a powered air-purifying respirator (PAPR), a disposable surgical cap, gown, gloves, and shoe covers when evaluating a laryngectomee with unknown, suspected, or positive COVID-19 status. Standard PPE, as defined by the Occupational Health and Safety Administration (OSHA), can be used for COVID-19-negative patients https://www.osha.gov/Publications/osha3151.pdf

It is recommended to defer nasopharyngoscopy and tracheoscopy if possible as these are high risk aerosol generating procedures. When performing flexible tracheoscopy, attempts should be made to minimize mucosal stimulation and resultant coughing.

A special article published by DrGivi and colleagues in JAMA Otolaryngology-Head & Neck Surgery, presented guidelines for head and neck physical examination and surgical and non-surgical procedures during the coronavirus (COVID-19) pandemic.

Because head and neck examinations are considered high risk in patients with suspected or confirmed COVID-19, the authors developed recommendations for health care workers based on review of the literature and communication with physicians with firsthand knowledge of safety procedures during the COVID-19 pandemic.

The guidelines stated that:

1. Non-urgent appointments should be postponed to limit infection of patients or health care workers. This may include postponing appointments for patients with benign disease and for those undergoing routine surveillance after treatment for head and neck cancer.

2. Patients should be queried by telephone about new or concerning signs or symptoms that may indicate recurrence and/or pending issues, as well as symptoms suggestive of COVID-19

3. In-person clinic visits should be offered to those at risk for significant negative outcomes without evaluation

4. Maintaining relationships with patients and support assessments that can be made without in-person examinations. The use of telephone, video, or telemedicine visits should be considered

5. In-person examinations should be limited to patients who need a thorough head and neck examination (e.g., postoperative visits, tracheoesophageal prosthesis complications, symptoms concerning for cancer recurrence, etc.). Detailed guidelines are provided for physical examinations and associated procedures

It is expected that following carefully planned routines and procedures, will enable providing adequate care and help protect the safety and health of health providers and patients.

To read the Guidelines click this link.
https://jamanetwork.com/journals/jamaotolaryngology/fullarticle/2764032

Hennessy et al. present the special considerations and best practice recommendations in the management of total laryngectomy patients. They also discuss recommendations for laryngectomy patients and how to minimize community exposures.

https://authorea.com/users/5588/articles/440471-a-commentary-on-the-management-of-total-laryngectomy-patients?commit=79a4762517151daa75e748822146d03e37328943

A review summarizing some of the more readily available clinical protocols for head and neck specialists caring for patients in an environment of a SARS CoV-2 mediated COVID-19 pandemic was published by Kowalski et al.
https://onlinelibrary.wiley.com/doi/pdf/10.1002/hed.26164

An international consensus published their recommendations for head and neck surgical oncology practice in a setting of acute severe resource constraint during the COVID-19 pandemic: https://www.thelancet.com/journals/lanonc/article/PIIS1470-2045(20)30334-X/fulltext

Chapter 8:

Making home Corona virus proof

How to coronavirus-proof your home

Staying at home as much as possible is recommended during the COVID-19 pandemic. However, making trips to the grocery store or pharmacy are necessary at some point.

Because recommendations for COVID-19 may change, monitoring one's local health department and the Centers for Disease Control and Prevention for updates is important.

It is best to designate a single person to be the household errand-runner to limit outside exposures. Setting up a disinfecting station in an area outside the home or in a room with low foot traffic where one can disinfect or leave packaged food can be helpful.

While being outside the home:

- Avoiding coming within less than six feet of others

- Wiping handles on carts or baskets while shopping

- Wearing mask at all times especially near other individuals

- It is not necessary to wear gloves. However, washing hands frequently while being out and avoiding touching one's face are important

When get back home

- Washing hands with soap and water for 20 seconds

- Disinfect takeout boxes and packaged foods at your disinfecting station

- Thoroughly wash produce before putting it in your kitchen

Disinfecting

- Disinfect everything touched - doorknobs, light switches, keys, phone, keyboards, remotes, etc.
- Using EPA-approved disinfectants (these include Clorox Disinfecting Wipes and certain Lysol sprays) and leaving surfaces wet for 3-5 minutes

Delivery

- Asking workers to drop deliveries off on the doorstep or an at a designated area
- If they need you to come to the door, keeping six feet of distance
- Paying and tipping online when possible
- After picking up mail from the mailbox, wash your hands
- Keep the mail and boxes for 1-2 days before opening. If this is not possible wash your hands after handling them

Laundry

- Washing clothes, towels and linens regularly on the warmest setting
- Disinfecting laundry hamper, too, or placing a removable liner inside it
- Not shaking dirty laundry to avoid dispersing the virus in the air

Guests

- Not allow guests over when social distancing is required

- When housing a family member or friend, avoiding shared living spaces as much as possible

- When they need to enter shared living spaces, keeping six feet of distance

If someone in the home gets sick

- First, consulting your doctor

- Isolating them in another room and asking them to use a separate restroom

- Disinfecting frequently touched surfaces every day

- Avoiding sharing items with them

- Wearing gloves when washing their laundry

- Continuing to wash hands frequently

- Asking them to wear a face mask if they have one

Supplies need

- EPA-approved disinfectants

- If one does not have disinfectants, making a bleach solution by mix four teaspoons bleach per quart of water; or using a 70% alcohol solution

- Laundry detergent

- Trash bags

- Prescription medicines (these can mail order)

- Canned foods — fruits, veggies, beans

- Dry goods — breads, pastas, nut butters

- Frozen foods — meats, veggies, fruits

Pets

- Supervising pet in the backyard

- Keeping distance from other humans when playing or walking with pets

- Asking someone in the household to take care of them while being sick

- When caring for pets while being sick, washing one's hands frquently

Sources of the information are:

Dr. Leana Wen, former Baltimore City Health Commissioner and an emergency physician and public health professor at George Washington University in Washington.

Dr. Koushik Kasanagottu, an internal medicine resident physician at John Hopkins Bayview Medical Center in Baltimore, Maryland.

Dr. Richard Kuhn, a virologist, director of the Purdue Institute of Inflammation, Immunology and Infectious Disease and editor-in-chief of the journal "Virology."

Centers for Disease Control and Prevention.

Addendum

Useful resources

- American cancer society information on head and neck cancer at:

  http://www.cancer.gov/cancertopics/types/head-and-neck/

- United Kingdom cancer support site on head and neck cancer at:

  https://www.macmillan.org.uk/information-and-support/larynx-cancer

- International Association of Laryngectomees at: https://www.theial.com/

- Oral Cancer Foundation at: http://oralcancerfoundation.org/

- Mouth Cancer Foundation at: http://www.mouthcancerfoundation.org/

- Support for People with Oral and Head and Neck Cancer at: http://www.spohnc.org/

- A site that contains useful links for laryngectomees and other head and neck cancer patients at: http://www.bestcancersites.com/laryngeal/

- Laryngectomee Newsletter by Itzhak Brook MD. COVID-19 management in laryngectomees https://laryngectomeenewsletter.blogspot.com/

- Head and Neck Cancer Alliance at: http://www.headandneck.org/

- Head and Neck Cancer Alliance Support Community at:

  http://www.inspire.com/groups/head-and-neck-cancer-alliance/

  The Thyroid, Head and Neck Cancer (THANC) Foundation supports research and education in the early detection and treatment of thyroid and head and neck cancer. https://thancfoundation.org/

- WebWhispers at: http://www.webwhispers.org/

- Self Help for Laryngectomee book by Edmund Lauder:

  https://www.inhealth.com/product_p/ta5000.htm

- My Voice - Itzhak Brook MD information Website at: http://dribrook.blogspot.com

- The Laryngectomee Guide by Itzhak Brook MD. Paperback and Kindle at

  http://amzn.to/150n3to Free download at http://www.entnet.org/content/laryngectomee-guide

- The Laryngectomee Guide Expanded Edition, 4th edition. by Itzhak Brook MD, Paperback and Kindle at https://www.amazon.com/dp/1795508299 Free download at

  http://bit.ly/38BJUnt

- Brook I. My Voice: A Physician's Personal Experience with Throat Cancer. Createspace, Charleston SC, 2009. ISBN:1-4392-6386-8   Paperback and Kindle at http://goo.gl/j3r51V Free download at https://dribrook.blogspot.com/p/my-voice-physicians-personal-experience.html

Laryngectomees groups in Facebook

- Laryngectomy Support

- Strictly speaking a laryngectomy

- Lary's speakeasy throat cancer group

- Survivors of head and neck cancer

- Throat and oral cancer survivors

- Head and neck cancer survivors

- Support for People with Oral and Head and Neck Cancer (SPOHNC)

- National Association of Laryngectomy Clubs (NALC)

- Webwhispers Facebook group

- Care givers for laryngectomees

List of the major medical suppliers for laryngectomees

- Atos Medical: http://www.atosmedical.us/

- Bruce Medical Supplies: http://www.brucemedical.com/

- Fahl Medizintechnik: http://www.fahl-medizintechnik.de/

- Griffin Laboratories: http://www.griffinlab.com/

- InHealth Technologies: http://store.inhealth.com/

- Lauder The Electrolarynx Company: http://www.electrolarynx.com/

- Luminaud Inc.: http://www.luminaud.com/

- Romet Electronic larynx: http://www.romet.us/

- Ultravoice: http://www.ultravoice.com/

- Ceredas : http://www.ceredas.com/

About the author

Dr. Itzhak Brook is a physician who specializes in pediatrics and infectious diseases. He is a Professor of Pediatrics at Georgetown University Washington D.C. and his areas of expertise are anaerobic and head and neck infections including sinusitis. He has done extensive research on respiratory tract infections and infections following exposure to ionizing radiation. Dr. Brook served in the US Navy for 27 years. He is the author of six medical textbooks, 160 medical book chapters and over 770 scientific publications. He is an editor of three and associate editor of four medical journals. Dr. Brook is the author of "My Voice-a Physician's Personal Experience with Throat Cancer", " The Laryngectomee Guide", and "In the Sands of Sinai-a Physician's Account of the Yom-Kippur War". He is a board member of the Head and Neck Cancer Alliance. Dr. Brook is the recipient of the 2012 J. Conley Medical Ethics Lectureship Award by the American Academy of Otolaryngology-Head and Neck Surgery. Dr. Brook was diagnosed with throat cancer in 2006 and became a laryngectomee in 2008.